Social Security Disability Benefits

How to Get Quick Approval

By James Stuart

Published by BizMove
www.bizmove.com

ISBN: 9781798402139

Table of Contents

1. Do You Qualify for Disability Benefits?   5

2. What is the Requirement for Work   7
   Prior to the Disability?

3. What is the Definition of "Disability"   9
   According to the SSA

4. How Does the SSA Determines   11
   That You Are Disabled

5. How Much Money Will You Get   13

6. How Long Will Your Eligibility for   15
   Benefits Last

7. What Can Cause Your Benefits To Stop   17

Special Bonus:

8. Sixty One Ways to Save Money   18

1. Do You Qualify for Disability Benefits?

Each month practically millions of Americans are getting thousands of dollars in disability benefits from the government. Why not you?

Once you read this book you'll know exactly whether you qualify for disability benefits and how to get a quick approval.

Once you get approved you'll start getting a check of up to $2500 each and every month for the rest of your life.

The first thing you need to find out is whether you qualify for disability benefits. Fortunately there are several online services that offer a free, no obligation Social Security disability eligibility evaluation. The best way to find out if you qualify is to use those free evaluation services, since they base their evaluation on your specific personal situation. I'm going to specify below what is required by the social security administration for a person to qualify for the benefits. Now even if you read this and think that you might not be qualified I still think that you should take advantage of the free evaluation offer, as they are experts and can find a way that you can qualify even if you don't see it at first glance.

According to the SSA To qualify for Social Security disability benefits, you need first to have worked in jobs covered by Social Security. Then you need to have a medical condition that meets Social Security's definition of disability. In general, they pay monthly cash benefits to people who are unable to work for a year or more because of a disability.

Benefits usually continue until you are able to work again on a regular basis, what if you can't work indefinitely? in this case you will get monthly checks for the rest of your life. There are also a number of special rules, called "work incentives," that provide continued benefits and health care coverage to help you make the transition back to work.

If you are receiving Social Security disability benefits when you reach full retirement age, your disability benefits automatically convert to retirement benefits, but the amount remains the same.

2. What is the Requirement for Work Prior to the Disability?

In addition to meeting their definition of disability, you must have worked long enough--and recently enough--under Social Security to qualify for disability benefits.

Social Security work credits are based on your total yearly wages or self-employment income. You can earn up to four credits each year.

The amount needed for a credit changes from year to year. In the time that this guide is written, for example, you earn one credit for each $1,160 of wages or self-employment income. When you've earned $4,640, you've earned your four credits for the year.

The number of work credits you need to qualify for disability benefits depends on your age when you become disabled. Generally, you need 40 credits, 20 of which were earned in the last 10 years ending with the year you become disabled. However, younger workers may qualify with fewer credits.

Side note: Remember that whatever your age is, you must have earned the required number of work credits within a certain period ending with the time you become disabled. If you qualify now but you stop working under Social Security, you may not continue to meet the disability work requirement in the future.

3. What is the Definition of "Disability" According to the SSA

The definition of disability under Social Security is different than other programs. Social Security pays only for total disability. No benefits are payable for partial disability or for short-term disability.

"Disability" under Social Security is based on your inability to work. The Social Security Administration (SSA) consider you disabled under Social Security rules if:

* You cannot do work that you did before;

* They decide that you cannot adjust to other work because of your medical condition(s); and

* Your disability has lasted or is expected to last for at least one year.

Does the above definition of "Disability" by the SSA seem strict and tough to comply with? Well, think again. The fact is that millions of ordinary people all across the United States are receiving disability money each and every month. In West Virginia, a whopping 9% of the population collects disability checks. In Arkansas, 8.2% are on disability, and in Alabama and Kentucky, 8.1%

collect disability. In Hale County Alabama 25% of the population receive disability checks, that's 1 in 4.

Now do you think that all these people fully comply word for word with the above "Disability" definition? Well, maybe they do or maybe they don't. The fact is that if a physician will determine that your backache disables you, this can lead to approving your application.

4. How Does the SSA Determines That You Are Disabled

To decide whether you are disabled, the SSA uses a process involving four questions. They are:

1. are you working?

If you are working and your earnings average more than $1,040 a month, you generally cannot be considered disabled (this number is applicable to the year in which this book has been written).

If you are not working, they will go to Step 2.

2. is your condition "sever"

Your condition must interfere with basic work-related activities for your claim to be considered. If it does not, they will find that you are not disabled.

If your condition does interfere with basic work-related activities, you go to Step 3.

3. is your condition found in the list of disabling conditions?

For each of the major body systems, the SSA maintains a list of medical conditions that are so severe they automatically mean that you are disabled. If your condition is not on the list, they have to decide if it is of equal severity to a medical condition that is on the list. If it is, they will find that you are disabled. If it is not, you then go to Step 4.

4. Can You Do the Work You Did Previously?

If your condition is severe but not at the same or equal level of severity as a medical condition on the list, then they must determine if it interferes with your ability to do the work you did previously. If it does not, your claim will be denied.

Special Situations

Most people who receive disability benefits are workers who qualify on their own records and meet the work and disability requirements I have just described. However, I want to point out some situations you may not know about:

* If You Are Blind Or Have Low Vision,

* If You Are The Worker's Widow Or Widower,

* Benefits For A Disabled Child,

* Disability Benefits For Wounded Warriors

5. How Much Money Will You Get

If your application is approved, your first Social Security benefit will be paid for the sixth full month after the date that the SSA find that your disability began.

Social Security benefits are paid in the month following the month for which they're due. This means that the benefit due for December would be paid to you in January, and so on.

The amount of your monthly disability benefit is based on your lifetime average earnings covered by Social Security.

Most SSDI recipients receive between $300 and $2,200. The average SSDI payment at the time of writing this book is $1,132. The maximum disability benefit at this time is $2,533.

When you start receiving disability benefits, certain members of your family also may qualify for benefits on your record. Benefits may be paid to your: spouse, divorced spouse, children, disabled child, and/or adult child disabled before age 22.

If any of your qualified family members apply for benefits, the SSA will ask for their Social Security numbers and their birth certificates.

If your spouse is applying for benefits, the SSA also may ask for proof of marriage, and dates of prior marriages, if applicable.

Each family member may be eligible for a monthly benefit of up to 50 percent of your disability rate. However, there is a limit to the amount they pay your family.

The total depends on your benefit amount and the number of family members who also qualify on your record. The total varies, but generally the total amount you and your family can receive is about 150 to 180 percent of your disability benefit.

If the sum of the benefits payable on your account is greater than the family limit, the benefits to the family members will be reduced proportionately. Your benefit will not be affected.

6. How Long Will Your Eligibility for Benefits Last

In most cases, you will continue to receive benefits as long as you are disabled. However, there are certain circumstances that may change your continuing eligibility for disability benefits. For example, your health may improve to the point where you are no longer considered disabled; or you would like to go back to work rather than depend on your disability benefits.

The law requires that the SSA review your case from time to time to verify that you are still disabled. You will be noticed if it is time to review your case, and they also will keep you informed about your benefit status. You also should be aware that you are responsible for letting them know if your health improves or you go back to work.

In general, your benefits will continue as long as you are disabled. However, the law requires that the SSA review your case periodically to see if you are still disabled. How often they review your case depends on whether your condition is expected to improve.

If medical improvement is:

* "Expected," your case will normally be reviewed within six to 18 months after your benefits start.

* "Possible," your case will normally be reviewed no sooner than three years.

* "Not expected," your case will normally be reviewed no sooner than seven years.

7. What Can Cause Your Benefits To Stop?

Two things can cause the SSA to decide that you are no longer disabled and to stop your benefits.

Your disability benefits will stop if you work at a level the SSA considers "substantial." In this time, average earnings of $1,040 or more per month are usually considered substantial.

Your disability benefits also will stop if they decide that your medical condition has improved to the point that you are no longer disabled.

According to SSA regulations you are responsible for promptly reporting any improvement in your condition, if you return to work, and certain other events as long as you are receiving disability benefits.

What if you are Interested in going back to work? There are special rules that help you keep your cash benefits and Medicare while you test your ability to work. This is called "work incentives." Work incentives include, but are not limited to, continued monthly benefits and Medicare coverage while you attempt to work on a full-time basis.

Special Bonus:

8. Sixty One Ways to Save Money

Here is a list of tips and ideas that will help you save money in various areas of your life:

Airline Fares

1.You may lower the price of a round trip air fare by as much as two-thirds by making certain your trip includes a Saturday evening stay over, and by purchasing the ticket in advance.

2.To make certain you have a cheap fare, even if you use a travel agent, contact all the airlines that fly where you want to go and ask what the lowest fare to your destination is.

3.Be flexible, if possible. Consider using low fare carriers or alternative airports and keep an eye out for fare wars.

Car Rental

1.Since car rental rates can vary greatly, shop around for the best basic rates. Ask about any additional charges (extra driver, gas, drop-off fees) and special offers.

2.Rental car companies offer various insurance and waiver options. Check with your automobile insurance agent and credit card company in advance to avoid duplicating any coverage you may already have.

New Cars

1.You can save thousands of dollars over the lifetime of a car by selecting a model that combines a low purchase price with low financing, insurance, gasoline, maintenance, and repair costs. Ask your local librarian for new car guides that contain this information.

2.Having selected a model, you can save hundreds of dollars by comparison shopping. Call at least five dealers for price quotes and let each know that you are calling others.

3.Remember there is no "cooling off" period on new car sales. Once you have signed a contract, you are obligated to buy the car.

Used Cars

1.Before buying any used car:

- Compare the seller's asking price with the average

retail price in a "bluebook" or other guide to car prices found at many libraries, banks, and credit unions.

- Have a mechanic you trust check the car, especially if the car is sold "as is."

2.Consider purchasing a used car from an individual you know and trust. They are more likely than other sellers to charge a lower price and point out any problems with the car.

Auto Leasing

1.Don't decide to lease a car just because the payments are lower than on a traditional auto loan. The leasing payments may be lower because you don't own the car at the end of the lease.

2.Leasing a car is very complicated. When shopping, consider the price of the car (known as the capitalized cost), your trade-in allowance, any down payment, monthly payments, various fees (excess mileage, excess "wear and tear," end-of- lease), and the cost of buying the car at the end of the lease. Keys to Vehicle Leasing: A Consumer Guide, published by the Federal Reserve Board and Federal Trade Commission, is a valuable source of information about auto leasing.

Gasoline

1.You can save hundreds of dollars a year by comparing prices at different stations, pumping gas yourself, and using the lowest-octane called for in your owner's manual.

2.You can save up to $100 a year on gas by keeping your engine tuned and your tires inflated to their proper pressure.

Car Repairs

1.Consumers lose billions of dollars each year on unneeded or poorly done car repairs. The most important step that you can take to save money on these repairs is to find a skilled, honest mechanic. Before you need repairs, look for a mechanic who:

- is certified and well established;

- has done good work for someone you know; and

- communicates well about repair options and costs.

Auto Insurance

1.You can save several hundred dollars a year by purchasing auto insurance from a licensed, low-price insurer. Call your state insurance department for a publication showing typical prices charged by different companies. Then call at least four of the lowest-priced, licensed insurers to learn what they would charge you for the same coverage.

2.Talk to your agent or insurer about raising your deductibles on collision and comprehensive coverages to at least $500 or, if you have an old car, dropping these coverages altogether. Taking these steps can save you hundreds of dollars a year.

3.Make certain that your new policy is in effect before dropping your old one.

Homeowner/Renter Insurance

1.You can save several hundred dollars a year on homeowner insurance and up to $50 a year on renter insurance by purchasing insurance from a low-price, licensed insurer. Ask your state insurance department for a publication showing typical prices charged by different licensed companies. Then call at least four of the lowest priced insurers to learn what they would charge you. If such a publication is not available, it is even more important to call at least four insurers for price quotes.

2.Make certain you purchase enough coverage to replace the house and its contents. "Replacement" on the house means rebuilding to its current condition.

3.Make certain your new policy is in effect before dropping your old one.

Life Insurance

1.If you want insurance protection only, and not a savings and investment product, buy a term life insurance policy.

2.If you want to buy a whole life, universal life, or other cash value policy, plan to hold it for at least 15 years. Canceling these policies after only a few years can more than double your life insurance costs.

3.Check your public library for information about the financial soundness of insurance companies and the prices they charge. The July 1998 issue of Consumer Reports is a valuable source of information about a number of insurers.

Checking

1.You can save more than $100 a year in fees by

selecting a checking account with a low (or no) minimum balance requirement that you can, and do, meet. Request a list of these and other fees that are charged on these accounts.

2.Banking institutions often will drop or lower checking fees if paychecks are directly deposited by your employer. Direct deposit offers the additional advantages of convenience, security, and immediate access to your money.

Savings and Investment Products

1.Before opening a savings or investment account with a bank or other financial institution, find out whether the account is insured by the federal government (FDIC or NCUA). An increasing number of products offered by these institutions, including mutual stock funds and annuities, are not insured.

2.To earn the highest return on savings (annual percentage yield) with little or no risk, consider certificates of deposit (CDs) and treasury bills or notes.

3.Once you select a type of savings or investment product, compare rates and fees offered by different institutions. These rates can vary a lot and, over time, can significantly affect interest earnings.

Credit Cards

1.You can save as much as a thousand dollars or more each year in lower credit card interest charges by paying off your entire bill each month.

2.If you are unable to pay off a large balance, pay as much as you can and switch to a credit card with a low annual percentage rate (APR). For a modest fee, RAM Research Corp. (800-344-7714) will send you a list of low-rate cards. You can obtain a list of low-rate cards by accessing "www.ramresearch.com.cardtrack" on the Internet.

3.You can reduce credit card fees, which may add up to more than $100 a year, by getting rid of all but one or two cards, and by avoiding late payment and over-the-credit limit fees.

Auto Loans

1.If you have significant savings earning a low interest rate, consider making a large down payment or even paying for the car in cash. This could save you as much as several thousand dollars in finance charges.

2.You can save as much as hundreds of dollars in finance charges by shopping for the cheapest loan. Contact several banks, your credit union, and the auto manufacturer's own finance company.

First Mortgage Loans

1.Although your monthly payment may be higher, you can save tens of thousands of dollars in interest charges by shopping for the shortest-term mortgage you can afford. On a $100,000 fixed-rate loan at 8% annual percentage rate (APR), for example, you will pay $90,000 less in interest on a 1 5-year mortgage than on a 30-year mortgage.

2.You can save thousands of dollars in interest charges by shopping for the lowest-rate mortgage with the fewest points. On a 15-year, $100,000 fixed-rate mortgage, just lowering the APR from 8.5% to 8.0% can save you more than $5,000 in interest charges. On this mortgage, paying two points instead of three would save you an additional $1,000.

3.If your local newspaper does not periodically run mortgage rate surveys, call at least six lenders for information about their rates (APRs), points, and fees. Then ask an accountant to compute precisely how much each mortgage option will cost and its tax implications.

4.Be aware that the interest rate on most adjustable rate mortgage loans (ARMs) can vary a great deal over the lifetime of the mortgage. An increase of several percentage points might raise payments by hundreds of dollars per month.

Mortgage Refinancing

1.Consider refinancing your mortgage if you can get a rate that is at least one percentage point lower than your existing mortgage rate and plan to keep the new mortgage for several years or more. Ask an accountant to calculate precisely how much your new mortgage (including up-front fees) will cost and whether, in the long run, it will cost less than your current mortgage.

Home Equity Loans

1.Be cautious in taking out home equity loans. These loans reduce the equity that you have built up in your home. If you are unable to make payments, you could lose your home.

2.Compare home equity loans offered by at least four banking institutions. In comparing these loans, consider not only the annual percentage rate (APR) but also points, closing costs, other fees, and the index for any variable rate changes.

Home Purchase

1.You can often negotiate a lower sale price by employing a buyer broker who works for you not the seller. If the buyer broker or the broker's firm also lists properties, there may be a conflict of interest, so ask them to tell you if they are showing you a property that they have listed.

2.Do not purchase any house until it has been examined by a home inspector that you selected.

Renting a Place to Live

1.Do not limit your rental housing search to classified ads or referrals from friends and acquaintances. Select buildings where you would like to live and contact their building manager or owner to see if anything is available.

2.Remember that signing a lease probably obligates you to make all monthly payments for the term of the agreement.

Home Improvement

1.Home repairs often cost thousands of dollars and are the subject of frequent complaints. Select from among several well established, licensed contractors who have submitted written, fixed-price bids for the work.

2.Do not sign any contract that requires full payment before satisfactory completion of the work.

Major Appliances

1.Consult Consumer Reports, available in most public libraries, for information about specific brands and how to evaluate them, including energy use. There are often great price and quality differences among brands.

2.Once you've selected a brand, check the phone book to learn what stores carry this brand, then call at least four of these stores for the prices of specific models. After each store has given you a quote, ask if that's the lowest price they can offer you. This comparison shopping can save you as much as $100 or more.

Electricity

1.To save as much as hundreds of dollars a year on electricity, make certain that any new appliances you purchase, especially air conditioners and furnaces, are energy-efficient. Information on the energy efficiency of major appliances is found on Energy Guide Labels required by federal law.

2.Enrolling in load management programs and off-hour rate programs offered by your electric utility may save you up to $100 a year in electricity costs. Call your electric utility for information about these cost-saving programs.

Home Heating

1.A home energy audit can identify ways to save up to hundreds of dollars a year on home heating (and air conditioning). Ask your electric or gas utility if they can do this audit for free or for a reasonable charge. If they cannot, ask them to refer you to a qualified professional.

Local Telephone Service

1.Check with your phone company to see whether a flat rate or measured service plan will save you the most money.

2.You will usually save money by buying your phones instead of leasing them.

3.Check your local phone bill to see if you have optional services that you don't really need or use. Each option you drop could save you $40 or more each year.

Long Distance Telephone Service

1.Long distance calls made during evenings, at night, or on weekends can cost significantly less than weekday calls.

2.If you make more than a few long distance calls each month, consider subscribing to a calling plan. Call several long distance companies to see which one has the least expensive plan for the calls you make.

3.Whenever possible, dial your long distance calls directly. Using the operator to complete a call can cost you an extra $6.

Food Purchased at Markets

1.You can save hundreds of dollars a year by shopping at the lower-priced food stores. Convenience stores often charge the highest prices.

2.You will spend less on food if you shop with a list.

3.You can save hundreds of dollars a year by comparing price-per-ounce or other unit prices on shelf labels. Stock up on those items with low per-unit costs.

Prescription Drugs

1.Since brand name drugs are usually much more expensive than their generic equivalents, ask your physician and pharmacist for generic drugs whenever appropriate.

2.Since pharmacies may charge widely different prices for the same medicine, call several. When taking a drug for a long time, also consider calling mail-order pharmacies, which often charge lower prices.

Funeral Arrangements

1.Make your wishes known about your funeral, memorial, or burial arrangements in writing. Be cautious about prepaying because there may be risks involved.

2.For information about the least costly options,

which could save you several thousand dollars, contact a local memorial society, which is usually listed in the Yellow Pages under funeral services.

3.Before selecting a funeral home, call several and ask for prices of specific goods and services, or visit them to obtain an itemized price list. You are entitled to this information by law and, by using it to comparison shop, you can save hundreds of dollars.

